Copyright © Stephanie Baker

All rights reserved. No part of this book may be reproduced, scanned or distributed in any printed or electronic form without permission. Please do not participate in or encourage piracy of copyrighted materials in violation of the author's rights. Purchase only authorized editions.

Chapter One

HEARTY LOW CARB MUFFINS

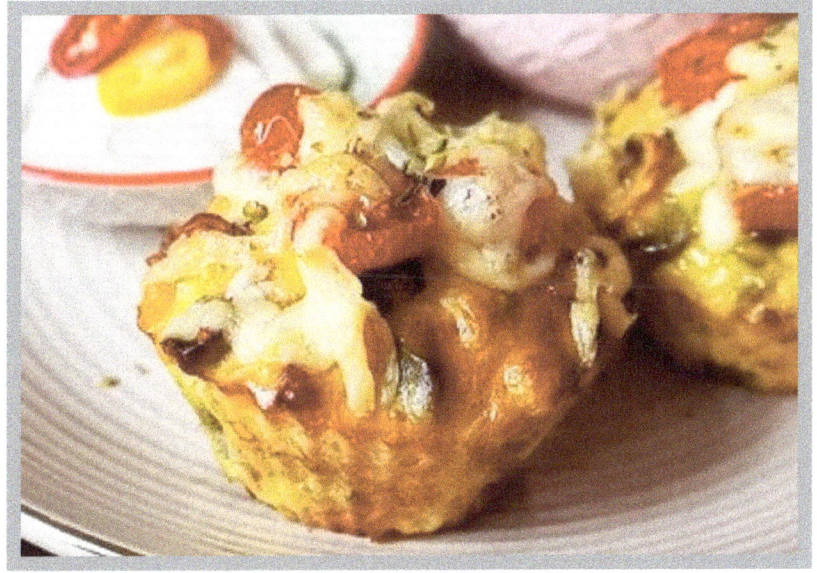

15 MINUTES.
Simple
852 kcal

. . .

INGREDIENTS

1 Servings

- 3 Egg (s)
- 50 g Gouda, grated
- 25 g Almond flour
- 1 Shallot (s), finely chopped
- 1 Spring onion (s), cut into small pieces
- 350 g Vegetables (peppers, mushrooms, cauliflower, peas, corn)
- N. B. Herbs
- Salt and pepper
- Butter

NUTRITIONAL VALUES per serving

kcal

852

protein

54.64 g

fat

57.24 g

Carbohydrate

29.21 g

PREPARATION

1. Approximate working time: 15 minutes
2. Approximate cooking / baking time: 30 minutes
3. Approximate total time: 45 minutes

4. Fry the onions in butter before adding the rest of the vegetables, which should be cut into small pieces. Season to taste with spices, salt, pepper, and other seasonings. I sometimes combine z. B. with curry, cumin, and paprika powder.
5. The eggs are then cracked and mixed with the Gouda and almond flour. This mixture has a strong "vegetable" flavor. If you don't like it as concentrated, simply add two more eggs, 75 g Gouda, and 40 g almond flour. Mix all together, pour into muffin tins, and bake for 30 minutes at 180 degrees top / bottom sun.
6. For the muffi, I used a 9-well silicone mold.

Chapter Two

LOW CARB VEGETABLE TUNA MUFFINS

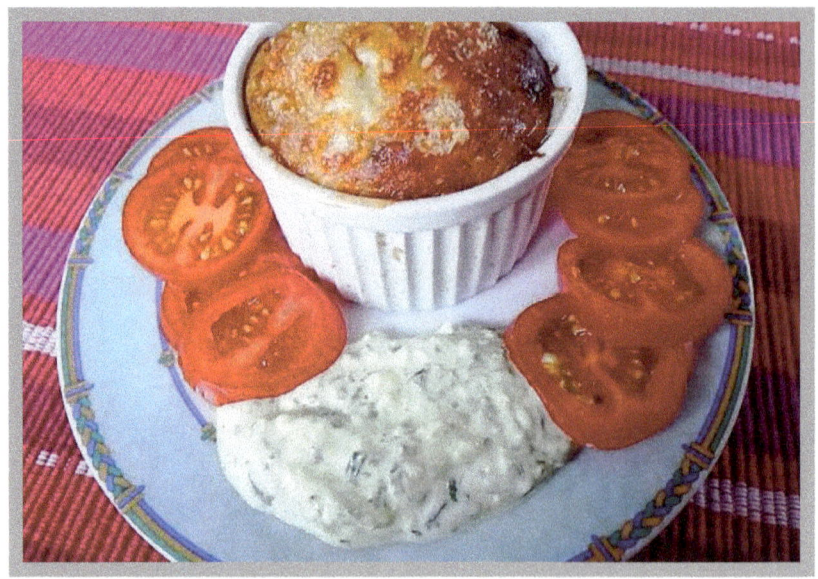

20 MIN.
simple
824 kcal

. . .

INGREDIENTS

2 Servings

- 1 can Tuna in its own juice
- 1 Egg (s)
- 200 gyogurt
- 200 gHerbal cream cheese
- 1 teaspoon Cream of horseradish
- 1 bunch dill
- ½ Bell pepper
- ½ zucchini
- 50 g Cheese, grated, e.g. Cheddar cheese
- 1 Onion (noun)
- Salt and pepper
- Paprika powder

Nutritional values per serving
kcal
824
protein
39.89 g
fat
68.05 g
Carbohydrate
13.63 g

PREPARATION

1. Approximate working time: Time: 20 minutes

2. Time to cook / bake: approx. Thirty minutes
3. Approximate total time: Time limit: 50 minutes
4. Shave the zucchini and cut it into very small cubes with a teaspoon. Break the peppers into small cubes as well.
5. In a large mixing bowl, combine the egg, crumbled and well-drained tuna, chopped dill, grated cheese, onion, bell pepper, and zucchini cubes. Season with paprika, salt, and pepper.
6. Fill the muffin liners with the tuna mixture (I've tried it with paper liners, but the paper will soak through).
7. Bake the muffins for about 30 minutes at 180 degrees Celsius.
8. Season with salt and pepper to make a dip with yoghurt, cream cheese, and creamed horseradish.
9. It goes well with a small salad.
10. Without the salad, the dish has about 16 g of carbohydrates per serving.

Chapter Three

LOW CARB COCONUT FLOUR MUFFINS

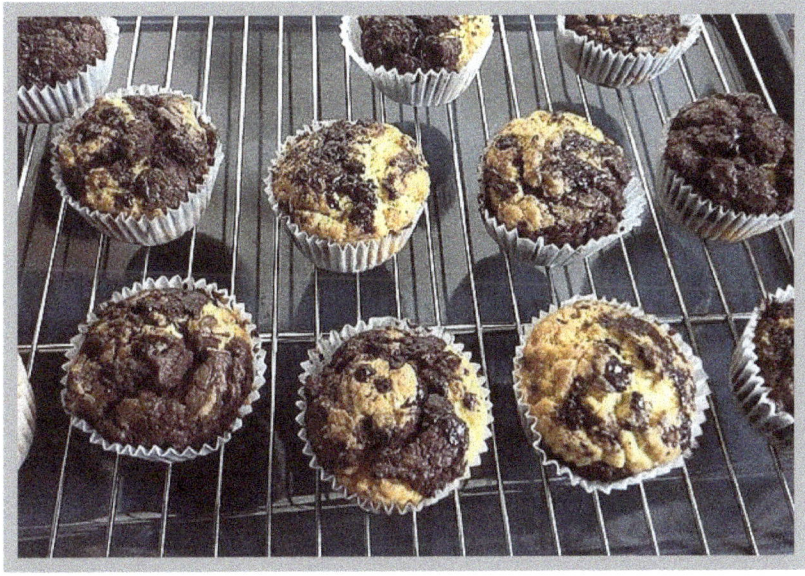

20 MIN.

simple
ingredients
1 Serving

- 125 g Coconut flour
- 80 g Erythritol (sugar substitute) (Xucker light), amount to taste
- 200 g Butter, Irish
- 4 large Egg (s), size L
- ½ tsp cinnamon
- ½ Lemon (s), the juice from it, with organic also like a bit of abrasion
- 1 bag / n Tartar baking powder or regular baking powder
- 6 tbsp Coconut milk or regular milk
- N. B. Baked cocoa, optional

POSSIBLY. Fat for the shape

INSTRUCTIONS

1. Approximate working time: 20 minutes
2. Approximate cooking / baking time: 30 minutes
3. Approximate total time: 50 minutes
4. In a mixing bowl, combine the coconut flour and erythritol. Mix all together with the mixer, including the butter, eggs, and the remaining ingredients.
5. The (coconut) milk is merely for consistency's sake. To get the traditional marble color, add baking cocoa to 1/3 of the dough.
6. Pour the batter into a muffin tin that has been greased or lined with paper liners. Now bake for 20 to 30 minutes at 180 degrees Celsius, depending on how brown you want them.

Tip: Since coconut flour binds a lot of moisture, the dough is very firm when made raw. Don't worry, I had to use the spoon to press the portions into the 12-cup muffin tin.

Allow the finished muffins to cool completely in the pan, as they are now very loose and prone to falling apart.

Chapter Four

LOW CARB MUFFINS

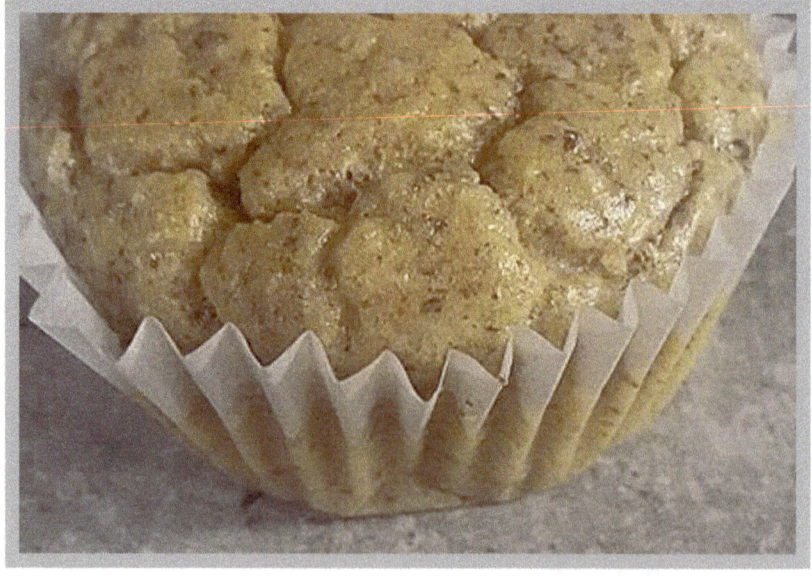

10 MIN.
   Simple
   2078 kcal

. . .

INGREDIENTS
1 Servings

- ½ Tsp salt
- ¼ tsp baking soda
- 200 g almond (s), ground
- 75 g margarine, or oil
- 4th egg (s)

N. B.SWEETENER

Nutritional values per serving
kcal
2078
protein
79.00 g
fat
190.27 g
Carbohydrate
15.64 g

PREPARATION

1. Approximate working time: 10 minutes
2. Approximate cooking / baking time: 20 minutes
3. Approximate total time: 30 minutes
4. Remove the eggs from their shells. Egg whites should be stiffened with a pinch of salt. For 1-2 minutes, whisk

together the egg yolks, margarine, and the remaining salt until frothy. Stir in the baking soda and ground almonds for a few seconds. To taste, change the amount of sweetener. Fold in the stiffly beaten egg white with care.

5. Fill 12 muffin tins or a springform pan with the batter. Bake for around 20 minutes at 150 ° C, lower and upper sun. You'll be safe if you use the stick test. Per stove heats up in a unique way.

Chapter Five
APPLE-BANANA MUFFINS, LOW CARB AND VEGAN

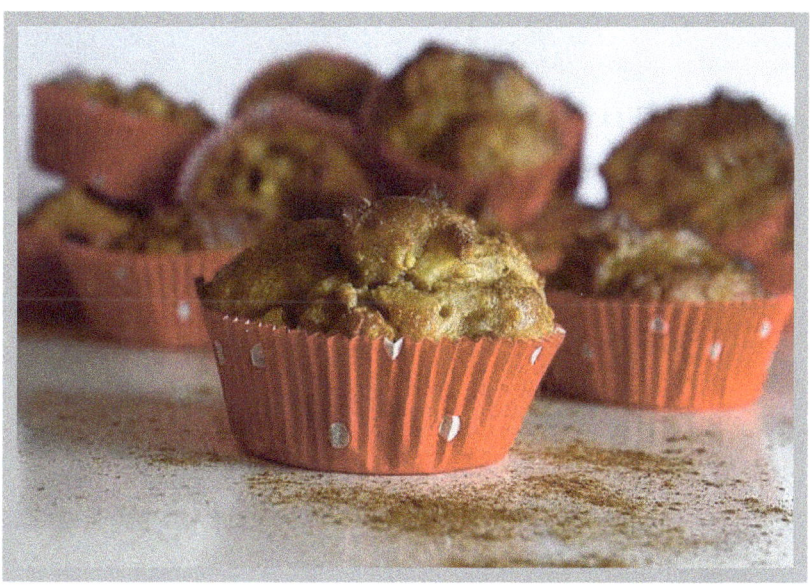

15 MINUTES.
Simple

. . .

INGREDIENTS

1 Servings

- 3 Banana (s), ripe
- 1 Apple
- 150 ml oil
- 100 gEgg white powder with vanilla flavor
- 50 g Coconut flour
- 50 g Flour (egg white flour)
- 50 g Coconut blossom sugar or xucker
- 1 pck.Baking powder
- 1 pck.Salt
- 1 shotMineral water

PREPARATION

1. Working time is about 15 minutes.
2. Time to cook/bake: approx. 25 minutes
3. Approximate total time: 40 minutes
4. Using a hand blender, puree the peeled bananas with the oil and sugar in a cup. After that, stir in the flour, baking powder, and salt. The dough would be really stiff. I added a splash of mineral water, which helps to loosen the bulk. The apple should now be cut into small cubes and folded into the batter.
5. Finally, spoon the dough into the muffin tins and bake for 20-25 minutes at 150° C in a preheated oven.
6. I like to sprinkle a little cinnamon on top of the apple and banana muffins before serving.

Chapter Six

HEARTY LOW-CARB MUFFINS

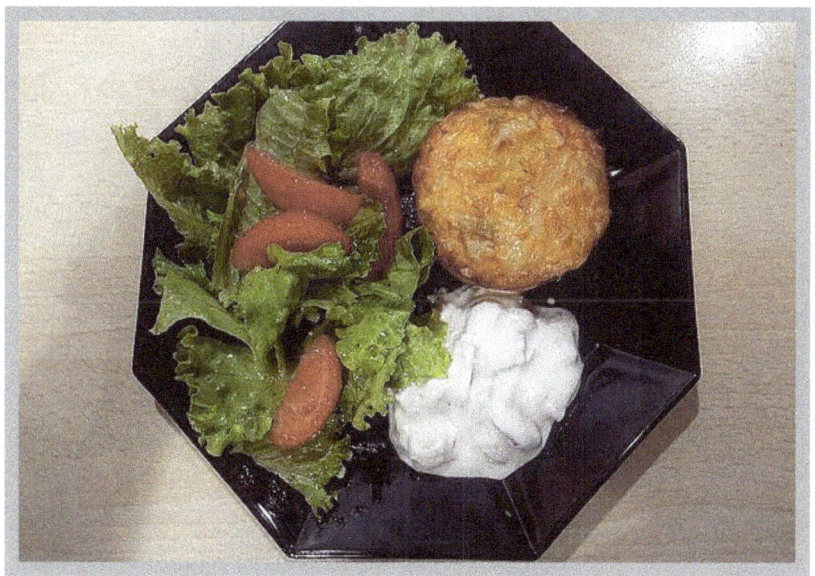

30 MIN.
　Normal
　418 kcal

. . .

INGREDIENTS

2 Serving

- 2 Egg (s)
- 100 gQuark (Fromage blanc)
- 50 g Almond flour
- 1 Spring onions)
- ½ Red pepper (s)
- 80 g Cheese, e.g. Gouda, Beaufort or similar, grated
- Somethingsalt and pepper
- SomethingPaprika powder
- Chili
- Something Fat for the molds

NUTRITIONAL VALUES per serving
kcal
418
protein
33.25 g
fat
28.53 g
Carbohydrate
6.55 g

PREPARATION

1. Approximate working time: 30 minutes
2. Approximate cooking / baking time: 30 minutes
3. Approximate total time: 1 hour

4. Preheat the oven to 180 degrees Celsius (convection).
5. Separate the eggs and beat the egg whites to a hard consistency. In a separate bowl, whisk together the almond flour, egg yolks, and quark.
6. If required, cut the spring onion into rings and the white into small cubes. Break the peppers into small cubes after peeling them. Combine the carrots, egg, and quark in a mixing bowl. 50 g of cheese should be added. Season with salt, pepper, paprika powder, and, if desired, chili powder.
7. Grease the muffin tins and fill with the batter. For two people, the sum given to me is 5 muffins. Bake for 25-30 minutes with the remaining 30 g of cheese on top.
8. The quality is similar to that of soufflé. The muffins may be eaten warm or cold, but they become firmer as they cool. This goes well with a salad and a dip (such as onion quark).
9. Non-vegetarians should add diced ham as well.

Chapter Seven

LOW CARB APRICOT CURD MUFFINS

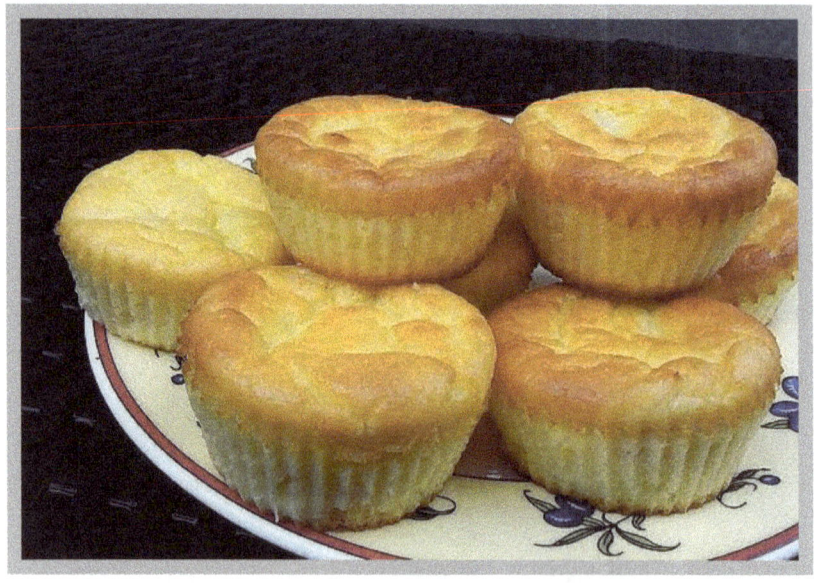

15 MINUTES.
   Normal

. . .

KETO MUFFIN

INGREDIENTS

1 Serving

- 30 g butter
- 60 g Erythritol (sugar substitute)
- 4 m.-large Egg (s)
- 250 gQuark, 20% fat content
- ½ Organic lemon (s), zest of it
- 1 teaspoon baking powder
- 1 pinch (s) salt
- 100 gGround almonds
- 100 gApricot

PREPARATION

1. Working time is about 15 minutes.
2. Time to cook/bake: approx. 25 minutes
3. Approximate total time: 40 minutes
4. Since the muffins can stick to paper liners, use silicone liners.
5. Preheat the oven to 180 degrees Celsius (350 degrees Fahrenheit) on the top and bottom racks. The apricots should be stoned and cut into small pieces.
6. To make the erythritol frothy, combine the softened butter and erythritol in a mixing bowl. Add the eggs one at a time, stirring well after each addition. Combine the quark and lemon zest in a mixing dish. Sift the baking powder and blend it with the quark, salt, and almonds in a mixing bowl. Fold in the sliced apricots with care.

7. Bake for about 25 minutes after pouring the batter into the molds.

Chapter Eight

LOW CARB MUFFINS

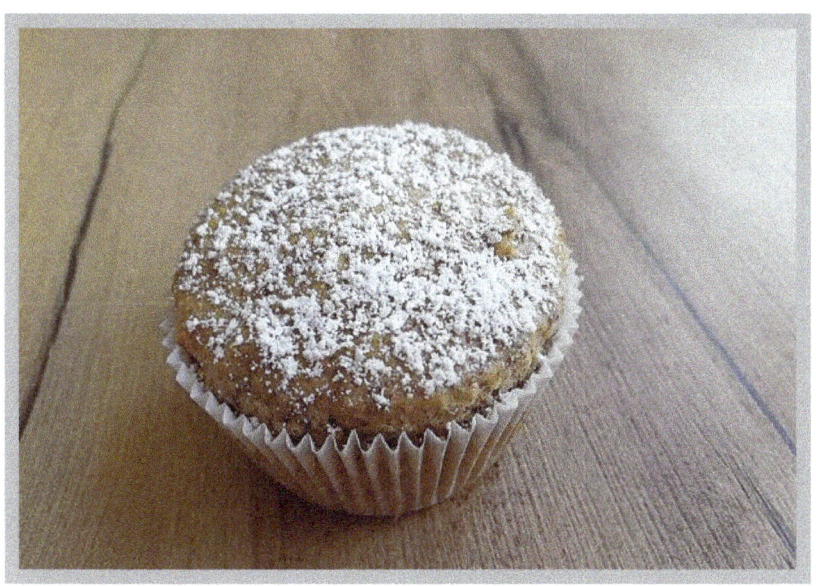

15 MINUTES.
Normal
179 kcal

. . .

INGREDIENTS

12 Servings

- 4th Egg (s)
- 1 pinch (s) salt
- 75 mlSunflower oil
- 200 gAlmond (s), ground
- ¼ tspBaking soda
- 5 tbspStevia, (sugar works too)
- 1 teaspoon Cinnamon powder

NUTRITIONAL VALUES per serving

kcal

179

protein

6.59 g

fat

16.56 g

Carbohydrate

1.52 g

PREPARATION

1. Approximate working time: 1 hour 15 minutes
2. Time to cook / bake: approx. Time: 20 minutes
3. Approximate total time: Time: 35 minutes
4. Remove the eggs from the shells. In a mixing bowl, whisk together the egg whites and salt until stiff. Combine the oil and egg yolk in a mixing bowl, then add

the remaining ingredients. Fold in the remaining egg whites after mixing in 1/3 of them. The dough is now placed in the molds. On the middle rack, bake for 20 minutes at 180° C.

VARIATIONS INCLUDE:

If desired, 2 teaspoons almond butter and 1 teaspoon Nutella may be added to the batter, or simply squeeze a few more sour cherries (approximately 3-5 per muffin) into the batter to make the muffins more juicy.

Chapter Nine

LOW CARB MUFFINS WITH YOGURT

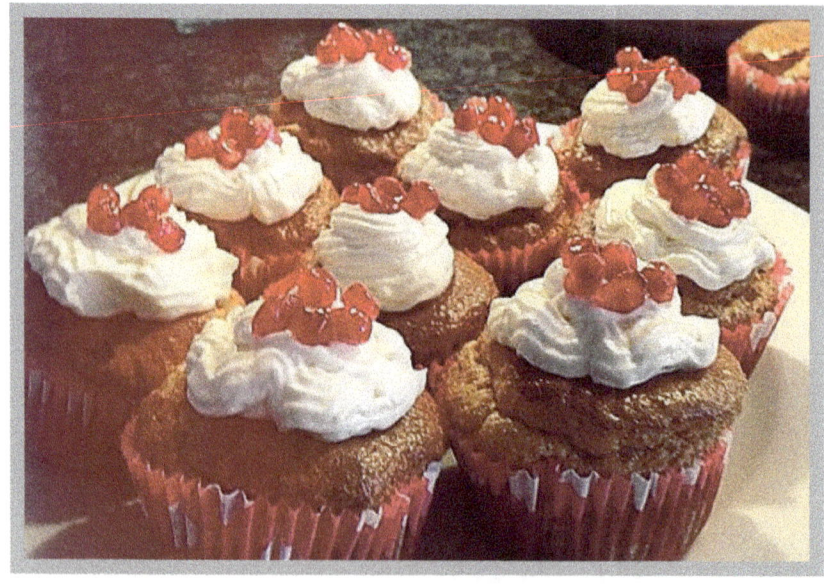

15 MINUTES.
Simple
2293 kcal

. . .

INGREDIENTS

1 Servings

- 3 Egg (s)
- 80 g Mascarpone
- 250 g Almond (s), ground
- ½ pck.Baking powder
- 150 g yogurt
- 3 tbsp Sweetener, liquid
- 1 pinch (s) salt

NUTRITIONAL VALUES per serving
kcal
2293
protein
92.97 g
fat
188.61 g
Carbohydrate
28.96 g

PREPARATION

1. About 15 minutes of work time
2. Approximate cooking / baking time: 20 minutes
3. Approximate total time: 35 minutes
4. Differentiate the eggs and beat the egg whites until stiff with a pinch of salt. After mixing the remaining

ingredients, gently fold in the egg white. Fill 12 muffin tins halfway with dough and bake for 20 minutes at 180° C. (make a stick test).
5. A single muffin contains about 1.5 to 2 g of carbohydrates and 200 calories.

Chapter Ten

LOW CARB CHOCOLATE COFFEE MUFFINS

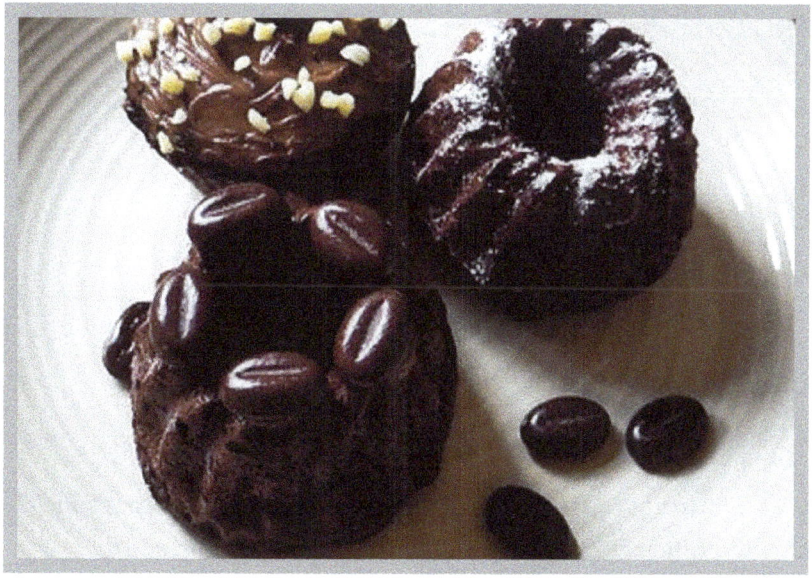

20 MIN.

Normal

. . .

INGREDIENTS

1 serving

- 100 g of dark chocolate with xylitol (Xukkolade)
- 80 g butter
- 100 g xylitol (sugar replacement)
- 4 egg (he), separated
- 2 Tl coffee powder, instant and
- 2 tablespoons water, hot or 2 tablespoons of strong coffee
- 200 g almond (s), ground
- 60 g of almond (s), chopped or almond leaves
- 1 Msp. Natron

INSTRUCTIONS

1. Working time is about 20 minutes.
2. Cooking/baking time is about 20 minutes.
3. Approximately 40 minutes total
4. With a pinch of salt, beat the egg whites until stiff and cold. Melt 100 g dark chocolate in a water bath. Combine 80 g butter and 100 g xylithite creamy in a mixing dish. Then add the egg yolks one at a time, stirring constantly. Then add about 2 tablespoons of solid coffee and the melted chocolate, stirring constantly.
5. 200 g milled almonds, 60 g chopped almonds, or a combination of almond leaves and a little soda, gradually integrated into the mass, but not all at once Fold in the egg whites last.
6. Fill muffin cups halfway with batter and bake for 20 - 25

minutes at 180° C top / bottom pressure. This is the time for a standard steel muffinback shape. It will take longer to scan the paper cups in the picture without the tin, which also scans a little more, which is why the stick sample was made.

7. Then, while they're still hot, take them out of the oven and drizzle them with rum. 1–2 teaspoons of Pro Muffin should suffice.

Chapter Eleven

LOW CARB CHERRY MARZIPAN MUFFINS

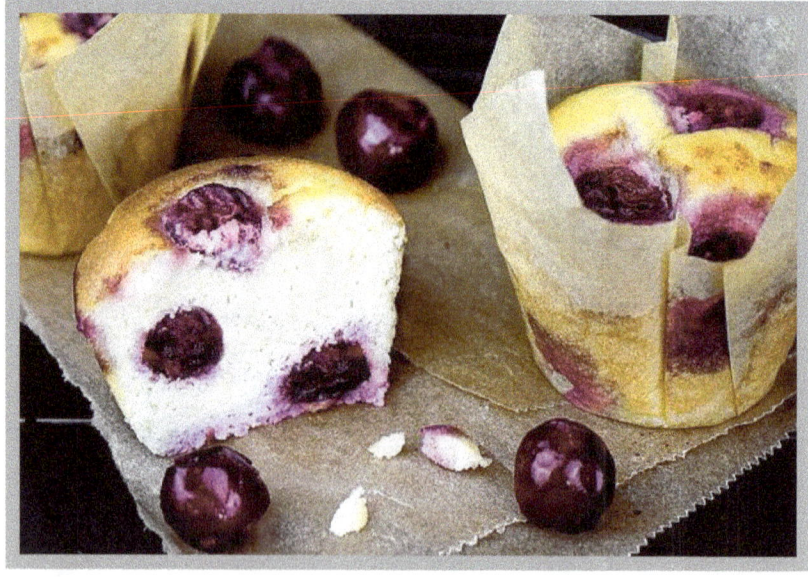

30 MIN.
   Simple
   180 kcal

. . .

INGREDIENTS
1 Servings

- 85 g Coconut flour
- 75 g Ground almonds
- 150 gXylitol (sugar substitute)
- 6th Egg (s)
- 75 g butter
- 100 gSour cherries, frozen, unsweetened
- 1 vialBitter almond flavor
- 1 teaspoon baking powder

PREPARATION

1. Approximate working time: 30 minutes
2. Approximate cooking / baking time: 30 minutes
3. Approximate total time: 1 hour
4. Preheat the oven to 175°C convection for 12 parts. Molds can be used to line the muffin tin.
5. In a mixing bowl, whisk together the eggs, xylitol, bitter almond taste, and butter until frothy. In a separate cup, combine the baking powder, coconut flour, and ground almonds, then stir them into the egg mixture. Pour the batter into the molds after folding in the cherries.
6. Preheat oven to 175°C and bake for 30 minutes.
7. Each muffin contains 180 calories.

Chapter Twelve

LOW CARB MARBLE CAKE

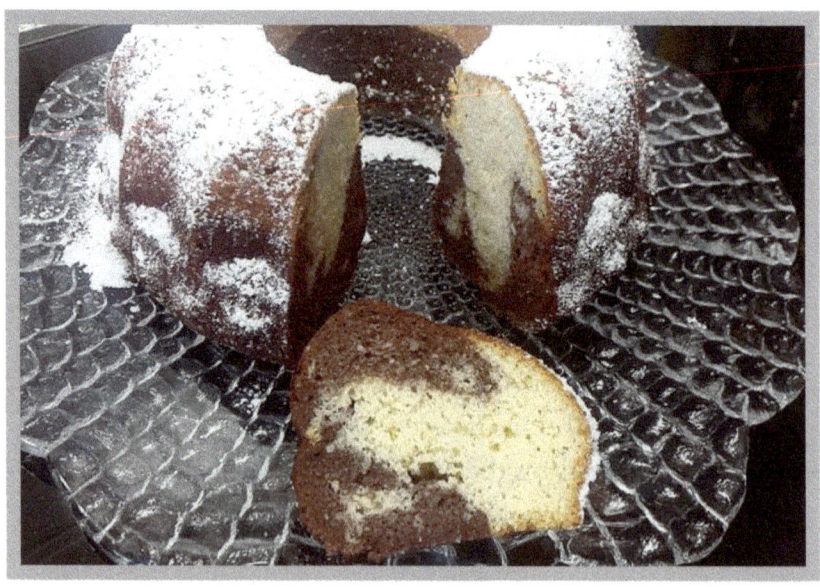

15 MINUTES.
Normal

. . .

KETO MUFFIN

INGREDIENTS

1 Serving
For the dough:

- 6th Egg (s), size M or L.
- 60 g Erythritol (sugar substitute)
- 50 g Xylitol (sugar substitute)
- 5 drops Stevia
- 50 gButter, room temperature
- 250 gQuark, 40% fat
- 1 pck.Bourbon vanilla flavor
- ¼ tsp, worked Tartar baking powder
- 1 tbsp, heaped Almond flour, de-oiled
- 1 ½ tbsp Coconut flour
- 190 gAlmond (s), ground, blanched
- 2 tbspBaking cocoa
- 1 pinch (s) salt
- ½ tspcinnamon
- Something Butter for the mold
- Almond (s), ground, for sprinkling the mold

PREPARATION

1. Approximate working time: 15 minutes
2. Time to cook / bake: approx. 50 minutes
3. 1 hour and 5 minutes is the estimated total time.
4. Preheat the oven to 160 degrees Celsius on the top and bottom racks. Brush a Guglhupfform generously with butter and generously sprinkle with ground almonds. To make the butter foamy, mix it with Xucker and Xucker

light, as well as stevia. Separate the eggs and blend the yolks with the butter mixture gradually. Stir in the quark, vanilla extract, almond flour, coconut flour, baking powder, and almonds until thoroughly combined. With a pinch of salt, beat the egg white until stiff. With a spatula, carefully raise under the batter until the egg whites are evenly distributed. Half of the batter should be poured into the mold. 2 teaspoons chocolate, carefully stirred into the other half of the dough with a spoon Place the dark dough on top of the light dough in the mold and fold the dark dough into the light dough with a fork. Smooth it out.

5. Place the pan in the oven on the 2nd rail from the bottom and bake for about 50 minutes at 160 ° C. Take a chopstick sample and put it in your mouth. Allow 15 minutes for the cake to cool in the tin. After that, remove the cake from the mold and cool fully on a wire rack. Powder Xucker should be sprinkled on top.
6. So far, everybody has enjoyed this moist cake.

Tip: If turning on the fan twice for 5 - 7 minutes each after the first 20 minutes of baking time isn't too much trouble for you, you can do so after the first 20 minutes of baking time.

Chapter Thirteen

LOW CARB MARBLE CAKE

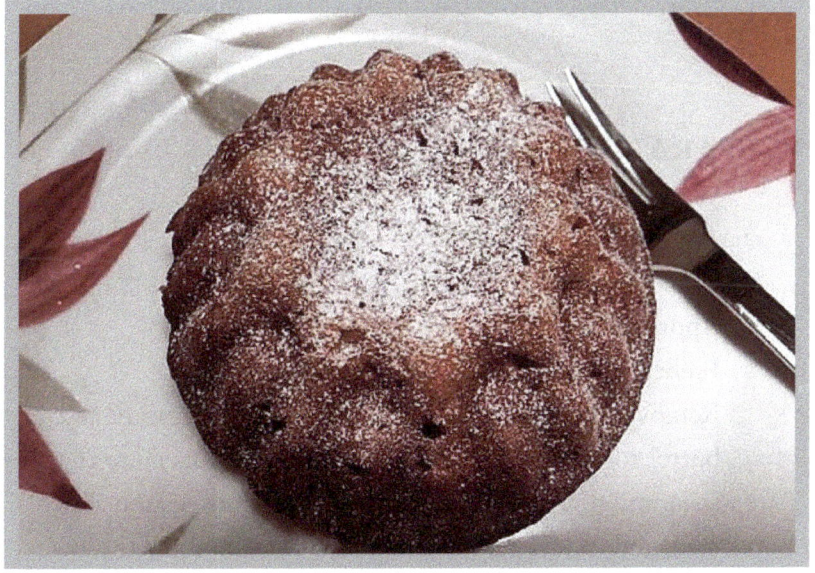

20 MIN.

Normal

INGREDIENTS

. . .

1 Servings

- 100 gXylitol (sugar substitute)
- 50 g butter
- 6ᵗʰ Egg (s)
- 250 gQuark
- Lemon zest
- Rum or rum flavor
- Vanilla pulp
- 200 gAlmond (s), ground
- 1 tbspAlmond flour
- 1 pinchbakin g soda
- 1 pinch (s) salt
- 1 tbspBaking cocoa

PREPARATION

1. Approximate working time: 20 minutes
2. Time to cook/bake: approx. 40 minutes
3. Approximate total time: 1 hour
4. Preheat the oven to 160 degrees Celsius.
5. Remove the eggs from the shells. Cream the xucker and butter together until smooth. Stir the egg yolks into the sugar mixture gradually. Combine the quark, lemon zest, rum, and vanilla pulp in a mixing bowl. Combine the ground almonds, 1 tablespoon almond flour, and a pinch of baking soda in a mixing bowl. Fold in the egg white, which has been stiffened with a pinch of salt. Create a half-dozen cuts in the dough. Half of the dough should be mixed with the sifted cocoa. You can, of course,

substitute fruit, nuts, or something else for the cocoa. Preheat oven to 160 degrees Celsius and bake for 40 minutes. Make a chopstick test in between checks.
6. The recipe makes enough for a regular loaf pan or a muffin tray; however, the baking time for muffins must be changed accordingly.

Chapter Fourteen

LOW CARB COCONUT HAZELNUT MUFFINS

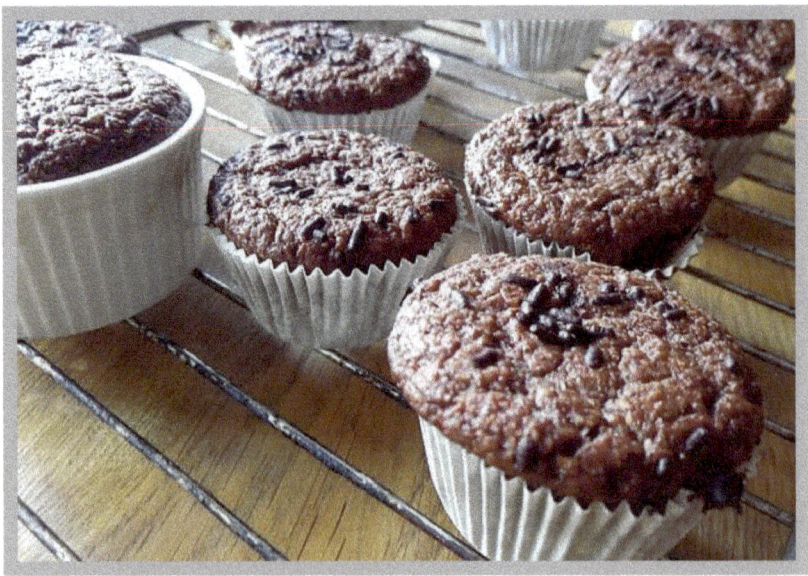

10 MIN.

Simple
INGREDIENTS
1 Serving

KETO MUFFIN

- 500 g low-fat quark
- 5 m.-large egg (s)
- 100 g desiccated coconut
- 125 g ground hazelnuts
- 100 g xylitol (sugar substitute), etc.
- 2 tbsp baking cocoa
- 1 pinch (s) cinnamon
- Something vanilla flavor or vanilla sugar
- 1 shot oil
- 1 pck. baking powder

TO SPRINKLE:
n. B. Chocolate sprinkles, dark

PREPARATION

1. Approximate working time: 10 minutes
2. Approximate cooking / baking time: 30 minutes
3. Approximate total time: 40 minutes
4. Preheat the oven to 175 degrees Celsius.
5. The amount of each ingredient varies. Add more desiccated coconut if you want it firmer to the bite, or more hazelnut flour if you want it nuttier.
6. In a blender, combine the dry ingredients first, then add the eggs, low-fat quark, and a splash of oil. You can use 1 to 2 spoons of coconut oil if you have some on hand. For 1 to 2 minutes, thoroughly combine all ingredients.
7. With a small spoon, distribute the mixture among the muffin cups. Keep an eye out because there will be some

leftovers. The muffins will grow by around half a cup. The molds can be almost fully filled to ensure a nice muffin top.

1. Preheat the oven to 350°F and bake the shape for 30 minutes. You can dress up the muffins by sprinkling dark chocolate sprinkles on top.

THIS RECIPE CONTAINS VERY few carbs, but plenty of healthy fats and protein. A delicious alternative to traditional muffins. The accuracy is excellent.

Chapter Fifteen

HAM AND CHEESE MUFFINS LOW CARB

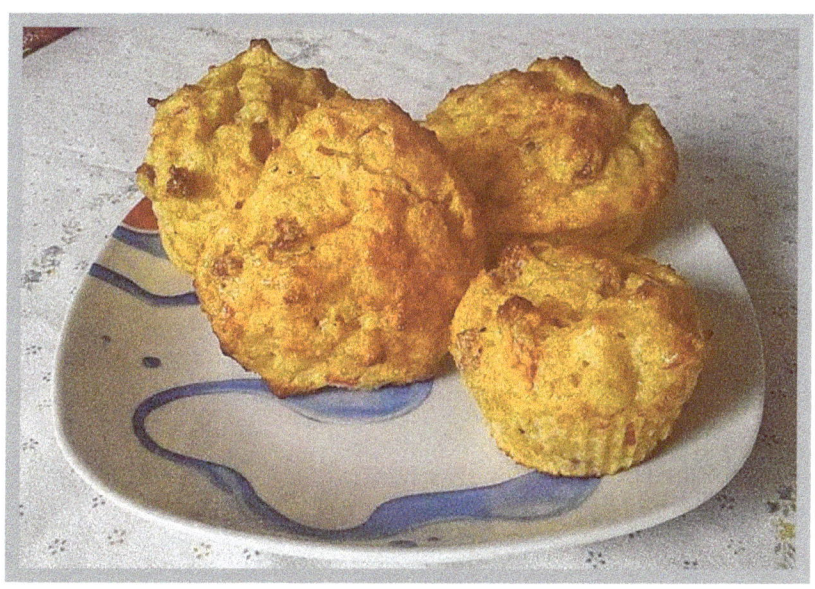

5 MIN.
   Simple
   1753 kcal

. . .

INGREDIENTS
1 Servings

- 500 glowfat quark
- 3 egg (s)
- 100 gham, smoked or cooked
- 250 gbran (oat or wheat bran)
- 100 gcheese, low fat, grated
- 1 teaspoon paprika powder
- 1 teaspoon baking powder
- Salt and pepper
- Possibly. Pepper (s) or leek or other vegetables, diced
- Possibly. Fat for the shape
- Possibly. Flour for the mold

NUTRITIONAL VALUES per serving
kcal
1753
protein
178.11 g
fat
76.28 g
Carbohydrate
83.09 g

PREPARATION

1. Approximate working time: 5 minutes
2. Approximate cooking / baking time: 20 minutes

3. Approximate total time: 25 minutes
4. Dice the ham finely. Vegetables can also be finely chopped and added, depending on your mood. I want it with paprika diced. Stir in the remaining ingredients thoroughly. Paprika powder, salt, and pepper to taste.
5. Fill silicone muffin molds or a muffin tray that has been greased and floured with the batter. Preheat the oven to 180 degrees Celsius and bake for about 20 minutes. Allow to cool slightly before removing from the molds and serving.

THE MUFFINS ARE delicious both cold and hot. It goes well with a salad.

Chapter Sixteen

CHOCOLATE MUFFINS WITHOUT FLOUR (LOW CARB)

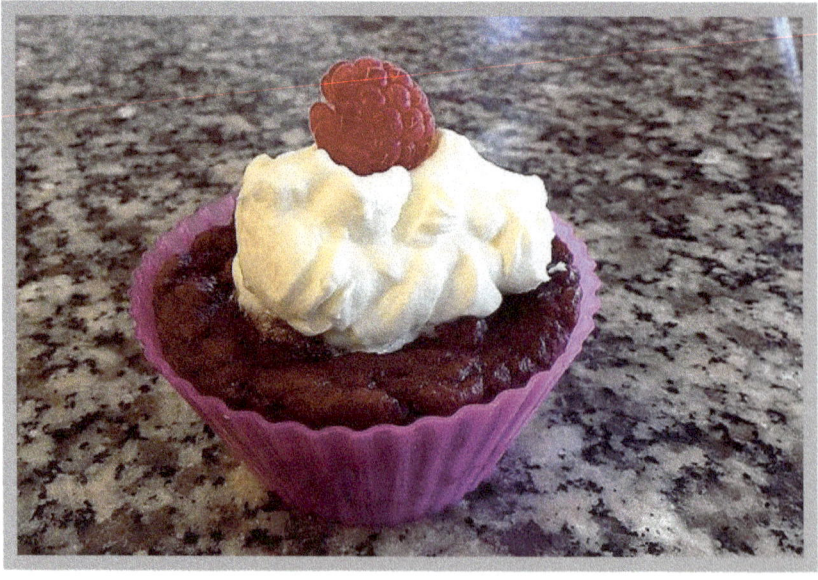

10 MIN.
Simple
812 kcal

. . .

INGREDIENTS
1 Servings

- 250 gCanned beans, red or white
- 3 Egg (s)
- 100 gQuark
- 2 tbsp.Cocoa powder
- 1 ½ tspbaking powder
- 70 g Raw cane sugar or stevia or sweetener
- Butter for the mold or paper liners
- For the topping:
- 50 mlcream
- 1 tbspQuark

n. B.sugar
n. B.Cherry

PREPARATION

1. Working time: approximately 10 minutes
2. Time to cook / bake: approx. 35 minutes
3. Approximate total time: 45 minutes
4. Preheat oven to 180 degrees Celsius. Deplete the beans and combine them with the eggs to make a puree. Then add the rest of the ingredients and stir to blend.
5. Pour the batter into a muffin tin that has been greased or lined with paper liners. Preheat oven to 350°F and bake for 35 minutes.
6. Made a topping by whipping 50 ml cream until stiff, then mixing in 1 tbsp quark and sweetening to taste. For the eye, add a cherry on top.

Chapter Seventeen
KIDAS LOW CARB VEGETABLE MUFFINS

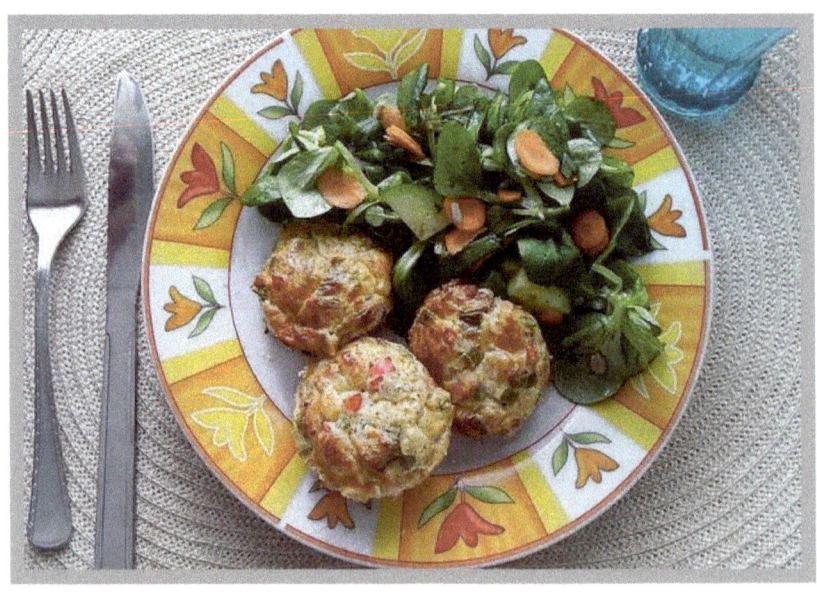

15 MINUTES.
Simple
1355 kcal

. . .

INGREDIENTS

1 serving

- 2 pepper (s)
- 100 g turkey grief section
- 3 spring onion (s)
- 150 g of lean quark
- 40 ml of milk
- 60 g of almonds, ground
- 50 g of cheese, grated
- 3 egg (he)
- 1 tablespoon of sunflower oil
- Margarine for greasing the muffin sheet

Nutritional values per serving
kcal
1355
protein
99.34 g
fat
95,10 g
Carbohydr.
25.20 g

PREPARATION

1. Working time is about 15 minutes.
2. Cooking/baking time is about 30 minutes.
3. Approximately 45 minutes total

4. Preheat the oven to 180 degrees Celsius with the fan on.
5. In a cup, cut the spring onions, paprika, and turkey sorrow into small pieces. Mix together the lean quark, milk, and ground almonds. Then stir in the grated cheese, eggs, and sunflower oil thoroughly.
6. Grease a ten-muffin sheet with margarine and fill to the rims with the batter. Preheat oven to 350°F and bake for 25–30 minutes.
7. It takes about 15 minutes to complete the mission.
8. It takes about 30 minutes to cook/bake.
9. Total time is around 45 minutes.
10. Preheat the oven to 180 degrees Celsius (350 degrees Fahrenheit) with the fan on.
11. Break the spring onions, paprika, and turkey sorrow into small pieces and place in a cup. Combine the lean quark, milk, and ground almonds in a mixing bowl. Then thoroughly mix the grated cheese, eggs, and sunflower oil.
12. Using margarine, grease a ten-muffin sheet and fill to the rims with the batter. Preheat the oven to 350 degrees Fahrenheit and bake for 25–30 minutes.

Chapter Eighteen

LOW CARB CHOCOLATE CINNAMON MUFFINS

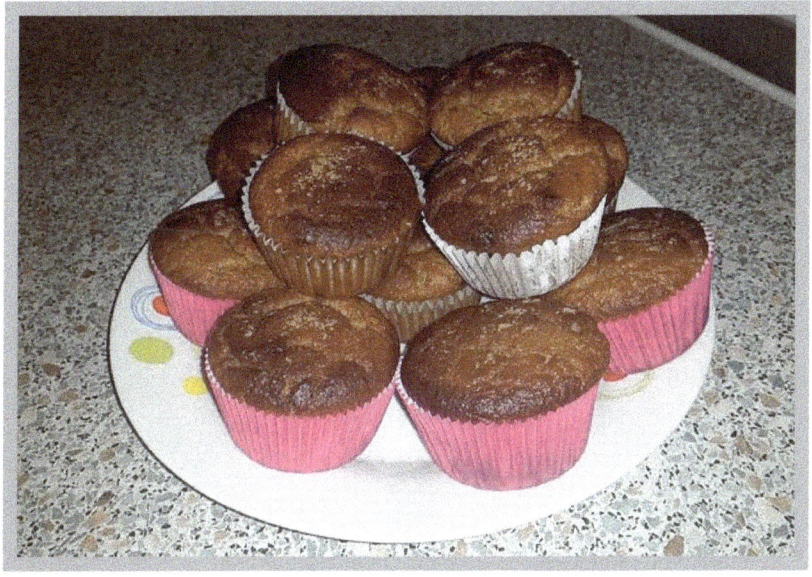

20 MIN.
Simple
2417 kcal

. . .

INGREDIENTS

1 Servings

- 50 g Chocolate decor (low carb chocolate drops)
- 3 Egg (s)
- 80 g lowfat quark
- 250 gAlmond (s), ground
- 1 teaspoonbaking powder
- 150 gyogurt
- 4 tbspSweetener (xucker)
- 1 pinch (s)salt
- 3 tsp cinnamon

Nutritional values per serving

kcal

2417

protein

102.72 g

fat

178.53 g

Carbohydrate

58.77 g

PREPARATION

1. Working time: approximately 20 minutes
2. Time to cook/bake: approx. 25 minutes
3. Approximate total time: 45 minutes

4. Separate the eggs and beat the egg whites until stiff with a pinch of salt.
5. In a mixing bowl, combine the chocolate drops, ground almonds, baking powder, xucker, and cinnamon.

1. In a separate bowl, combine the low-fat quark and yogurt. Now add the dry ingredients and stir for about 2 minutes with a mixer. Lastly, fold in the egg whites. Fill a muffin tin to the brim with batter and line with paper liners.
2. Preheat the oven to 180 degrees Celsius and bake for 25 minutes.

Chapter Nineteen

BASIC RECIPE FOR LOW-CARB MUFFINS

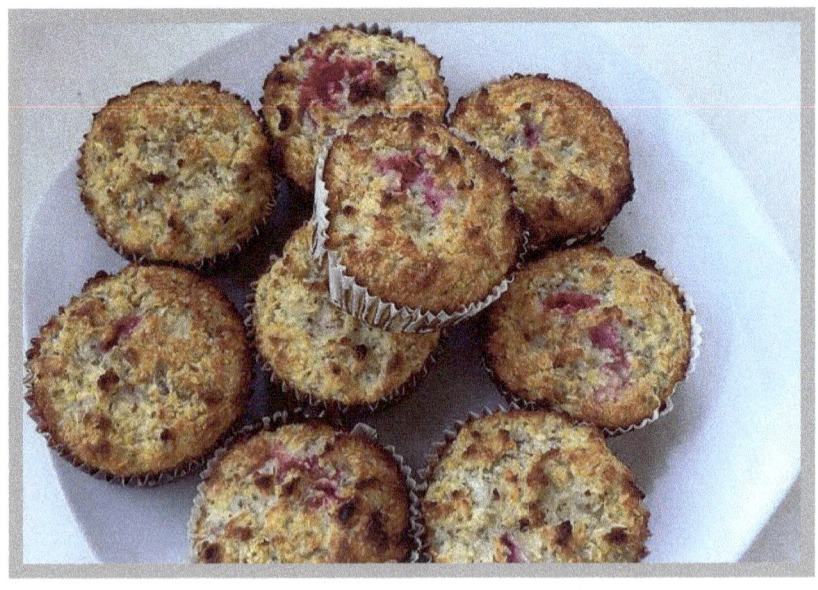

15 MINUTES.
Simple
1680 kcal

· · ·

INGREDIENTS

1 Servings

- 80 g Almond (s), blanched, ground
- 50 g Desiccated coconut
- 1 tbsp baking powder
- 2 Egg (s)
- 5 tbsp Coconut oil
- 5 tbsp Coconut milk
- 3 tbsp Natural yogurt, low-fat
- ½ Lemon (s) or orange, the juice of it
- 3 tsp Honey or agave syrup or maple syrup

NUTRITIONAL VALUES per serving

kcal
1680
protein
45.78 g
fat
151.08 g
Carbohydrate
38.59 g

PREPARATION

1. Working time is about 15 minutes.
2. Approximate cooking / baking time: 20 minutes
3. Approximate total time: 35 minutes
4. To make the eggs frothy, whisk them together until they

are light and fluffy. Toss the eggs with the moist ingredients (oil, coconut milk, cream, lemon or orange juice, honey). In a separate bowl, combine the dry ingredients (almonds, desiccated coconut, baking powder), then add to the liquid mixture.

5. Carefully mix all of the ingredients so they form a homogeneous mass. Fill the molds halfway with dough and bake for 15 to 20 minutes at 175° C top / bottom pressure.
6. You can also add chocolate, vanilla, cinnamon, fruits, or something else you want if you want.

Chapter Twenty
LOW-CARB MUFFINS WITH STEVIA

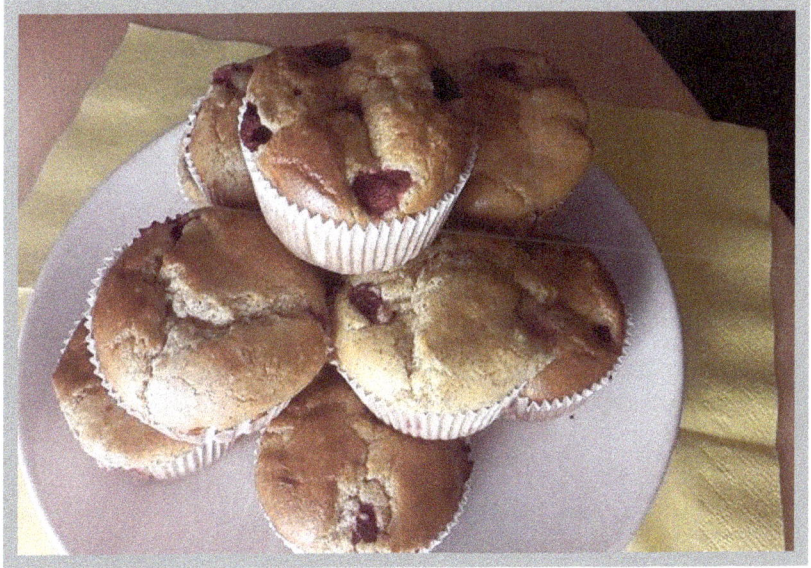

10 MIN.
Simple
2280 kcal

. . .

INGREDIENTS
1 Servings

- 4^(th) Egg (s), separated
- 1 pinch (s) salt
- 150 glowfat quark
- 75 mloil
- 4 tspStevia powder
- 200 gGround almonds
- 1 teaspoon Cinnamon powder
- 1 teaspoon baking powder

n. B.Raspberries or cherries

NUTRITIONAL VALUES per serving
kcal
2280
protein
99.97 g
fat
199.15 g
Carbohydrate
26.63 g

PREPARATION

1. Working time: approximately 10 minutes
2. Time to cook/bake: approx. 25 minutes
3. Approximate total time: 35 minutes
4. Using an electric mixer, stiffen the egg whites. Combine

KETO MUFFIN

the egg yolks, salt, stevia, oil, and quark in a frothy mixture. Combine the ground almonds, baking powder, and cinnamon in a mixing bowl. Fold in the egg whites with care.

5. Fill the wells of a 12-cup muffin pan with the mixture. 3–5 raspberries or cherries should be pressed into the mixture. Bake for 25 - 30 minutes at 170° C (top / bottom heat).

Chapter Twenty-One
BLUEBERRY CHOCOLATE MUFFINS LOW CARB

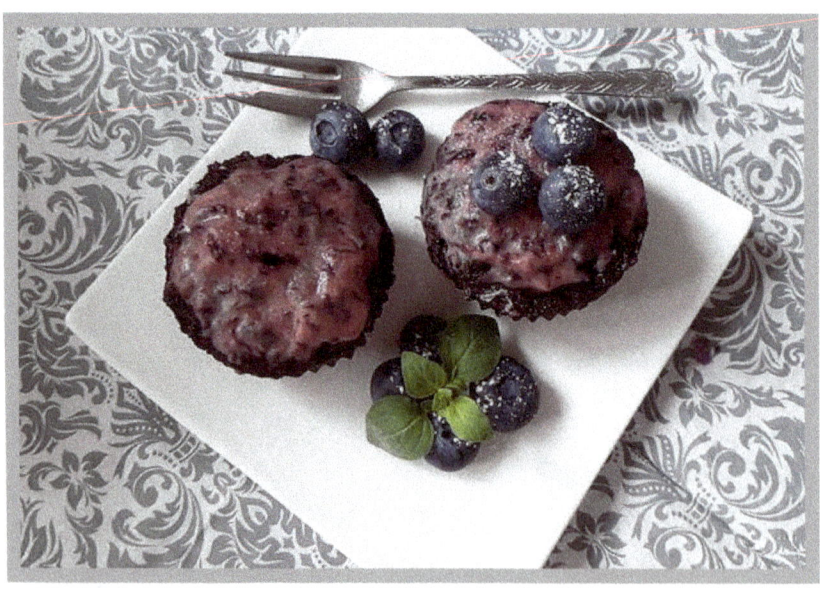

10 MIN.

Normal

915 kcal

. . .

INGREDIENTS

1 Servings
For the dough:

- 100 gzucchini
- 2 egg (s), size l
- 40 gerythritol (sugar substitute)
- 1 teaspoon baking powder
- 20 g baking cocoa
- 100 gground almonds
- 1 teaspoonprotein powder, chocolate
- 90 gblueberries

For the topping:

- 35 gblueberries
- 4 tbspErythritol (powdered sugar substitute)

Nutritional values per serving
kcal
915
protein
50.44 g
fat
69.88 g
Carbohydrate
21.58 g

PREPARATION

1. Approximate working time: 10 minutes
2. Time to cook/bake: approx. 25 minutes
3. Approximate total time: 35 minutes
4. To make the dough, finely grind the zucchini and combine it with all of the other ingredients (except the blueberries) in a hand mixer. Divide the batter into muffin silicone molds after folding in the blueberries. Bake the muffins for 20-25 minutes at 180°C (stick test), then cool completely before carefully removing them from the molds.
5. To make the topping, use a magic wand to puree the blueberries and then whisk in enough powdered sugar until it has a smooth consistency. 4 tbsp was all I wanted. Then, using a silicone brush, spread the mixture on the muffins.
6. Refrigerate the muffins after making them. They're a perfect, juicy summer treat when they're chilled.
7. I was able to fill 9 muffin tins with the dough, giving each muffin about 110 calories and 2.5 grams of fat.

Chapter Twenty-Two

LOW CARB CHOCOLATE MUFFINS WITH COCONUT OIL

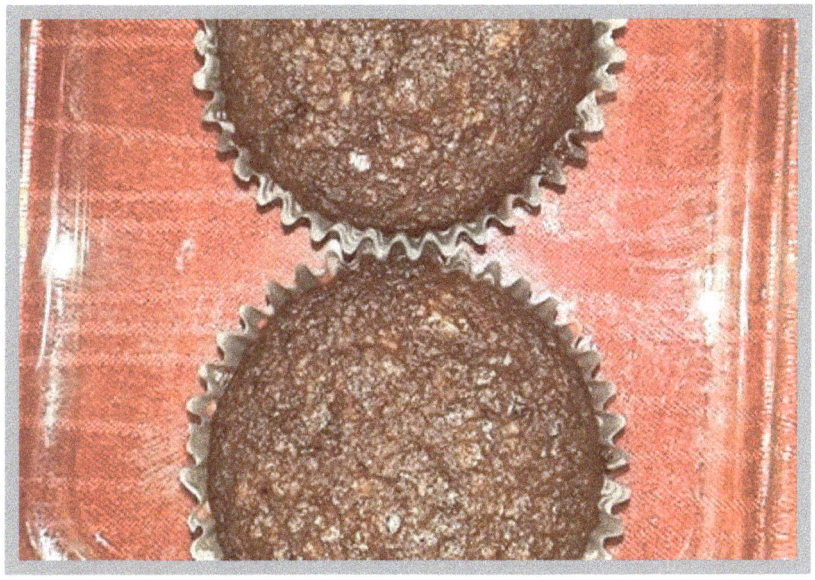

10 MIN.

Normal

. . .

INGREDIENTS

1 Servings

- 3 Egg (s)
- 70 g Ground almonds
- 60 g Coconut oil, alternatively butter
- 1 teaspoon baking powder
- 1 pinch (s)salt
- 2 tbsp, heaped Xylitol (sugar substitute)
- 2 tbsp, heaped Cocoa powder
- 1 tbsp Almonds, chopped
- 2 tbsp Walnut kernels, chopped
- Something Bitter almond oil, to taste

PREPARATION

1. Working time: approximately 10 minutes
2. Approximate cooking / baking time: 20 minutes
3. Approximate total time: 30 minutes
4. Preheat the oven to 170 degrees Celsius.
5. In a saucepan, melt the coconut oil. Separate the eggs and use the whisk to whip the egg whites.
6. Slowly drizzle in the coconut oil when whisking the egg yolks.
7. Combine the remaining ingredients and stir well. Finally, fold in the egg whites and put the mixture in muffin cups.
8. The batter can make 6 big muffins. I use muffin tins and paper liners.

9. After baking, leave the muffins in the oven to cool for 15-20 minutes with the oven door slightly ajar.

Chapter Twenty-Three
LOW CARB SOY MUFFINS

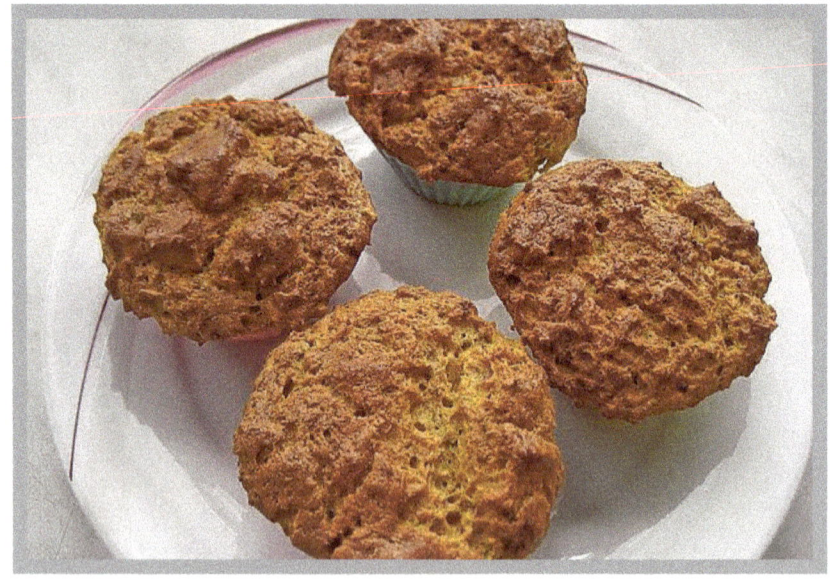

30 MIN.
Simple
475 kcal

. . .

INGREDIENTS

1 Serving

- 80 g Soy flour, defatted
- 100 glowfat quark
- 3 protein
- 1 egg yolk
- 1 pinch (s) Herbs of choice, chopped
- 1 pinch (s) salt
- 1 teaspoon, heapedBaking soda

Nutritional values per serving

kcal

475

protein

60.40 g

fat

22.75 g

Carbohydrate

4.35 g

PREPARATION

1. Working time is about 30 minutes.
2. Approximate total time: 30 minutes
3. Combine the soy flour and baking soda in a mixing bowl. Cream together the egg yolks, quark, salt, and herbs (I personally added some parsley and basil). Using an electric mixer, stiffen the egg whites. Gradually pour the

soy flour into the egg yolk mixture through a sieve. Fold in the egg whites with care. Fill muffin tins halfway with the batter.

4. Bake for 30 minutes at 160 degrees Celsius in a preheated oven, then for another 14 minutes at 100 degrees Celsius.
5. With the necessary addition of cinnamon and fruit, the recipe can also be turned into a sweet muffin version. There's no visual difference between these and "normal" muffins!

Chapter Twenty-Four

LOW CARB CAULIFLOWER MUFFINS

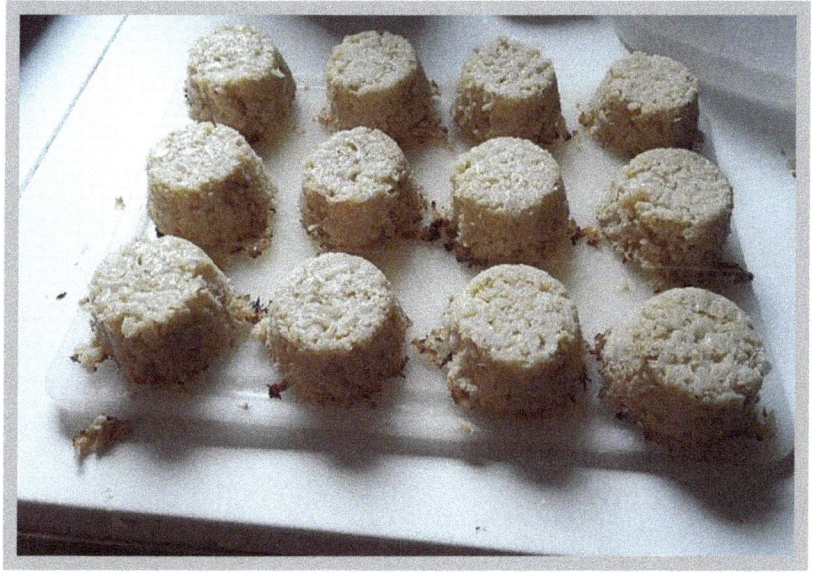

20 MIN.

Simple

781 kcal

. . .

INGREDIENTS

1 Serving

- 400 gcauliflower
- 1 Egg (s)
- 1 teaspoon Vegetable broth powder
- 150 gCheddar cheese, grated
- 1 m.-large Onion (noun)
- 1 Garlic cloves)
- 1 pinch (s) salt
- 1 pinch (s) pepper

Nutritional values per serving

kcal

781

protein

54.57 g

fat

55.87 g

Carbohydrate

14.34 g

PREPARATION

1. Approximate working time: Time: 20 minutes
2. Time to cook / bake: approx. Time: 40 minutes
3. Approximate total time: a single hour
4. Cook the cauliflower until it is tender but not too soft, roughly chopped. It can also be microwaved for 8

minutes at 800 W in a suitable saucepan with 2 teaspoons of water.
5. Then, using a potato masher, finely cut the cauliflower. A meat grinder or a hand blender may also be used. Make sure the cauliflower is fully drained. Remove the liquid in a salad spinner if possible. It's also possible to wring out the water with a clean kitchen towel.
6. Combine the cauliflower, cheese, grated cheddar, finely chopped onion, and garlic in a large mixing bowl.
7. Oil the muffin tin by spraying or brushing it. Make the vegetable broth and pour it into the muffin tins, making sure the bottoms of each hole are well covered. Fill the mold with the cauliflower mixture and smooth it out.
8. Preheat oven to 180 degrees Celsius and bake for 30 to 40 minutes.
9. Allow to cool slightly before removing the muffins and serving. It's also healthy cold.

VARIATIONS: As a low-calorie and low-carbohydrate side dish, omit the cheese. Other types of cheese, such as Parmesan and Emmentaler, are also delicious, particularly when served hot with chili.

150 calories and 8 grams of potassium per muffin; without cheese, 40 calories and 7 grams of potassium.

Chapter Twenty-Five

FLOURLESS LOW CARB MUFFINS WITH FRESH HERBS

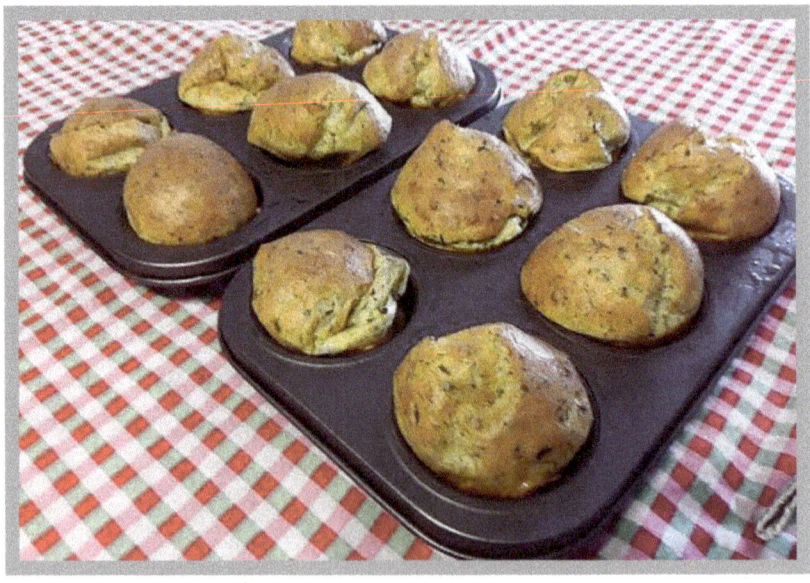

5 MIN.

Simple

. . .

KETO MUFFIN

INGREDIENTS
1 Serving

- 250 glowfat quark
- 4 m.-large Egg (s)
- 9 tbsp Egg substitute powder, low in protein, e.g. from hammer mill
- 1 bag / n baking powder
- 1 pck. 8 herbs, frozen, approx. 50 g
- 1 tbsp, heaped Dill, freshly chopped
- 2 pinch (s) Salt and pepper, whiter

PREPARATION

1. Approximate working time: 5 minutes
2. Approximate rest time: 10 minutes
3. Time to cook / bake: approx. 35 minutes
4. Approximate total time: 50 minutes
5. In a mixing bowl, whisk together the eggs and add the remaining ingredients. With a kitchen mixer, combine all of the ingredients until they are evenly homogeneous.
6. In the wells of a 12 mafin mold, spread the milk.
7. Slide the muffin tray onto the middle rack of an oven preheated to 180 ° C top / bottom heat and bake the muffins for 30 - 35 minutes, until browned.
8. Remove the tray from the oven and set it aside to cool.
9. When fried, the muffins would not become crispy. These are eaten fresh baked for breakfast or dinner, topped with herbal quark or fresh cold cuts, as an accompaniment to meat and egg salads.

Chapter Twenty-Six
LOWCARB MUFFINS WITH BERRIES

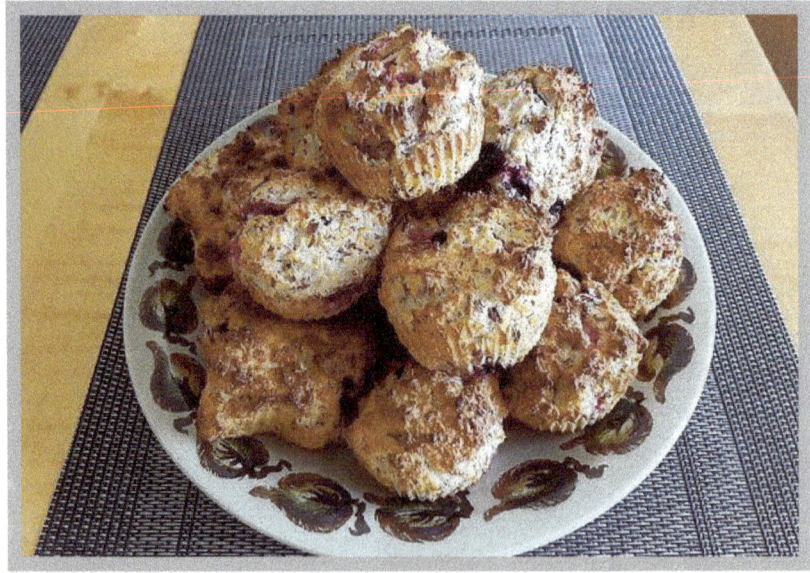

10 MIN.
   Simple
   200 kcal

. . .

INGREDIENTS

1 Serving

- 50 g Almond (s), ground
- 50 g Desiccated coconut
- 25 g Flaxseed, broken or whole
- 2 tbsp Soy flour, about 12 g
- 1 pinch (s) salt
- 1 teaspoon baking powder
- 30 g Butter, soft
- 100 g Quark, 20% fat
- 2 Egg (s)
- 30 g Blackberries, frozen or fresh
- 30 g Blueberries, frozen or fresh
- 1 teaspoon Sweetener, liquid, or other sweetener of your choice
- 4 tbsp water

PREPARATION

1. Working time: approximately 10 minutes
2. Time to cook / bake: approx. 15 minutes
3. Approximate total time: 25 minutes
4. Preheat the oven to 175 degrees Celsius. Grease the muffin tin and set aside. It's difficult to keep the paper cases off the muffins!
5. Mix the dry ingredients well in a mixing bowl, making sure there are no lumps. Stir in the softened butter, eggs, and quark. Add the sweetener and water, then fold in the berries carefully.

6. Bake for 15-20 minutes after pouring the batter into the molds.
7. When you can't see scrambled eggs any longer, this is the dish to make. The almonds, desiccated coconut, and flax seeds give the muffins a light "cereal-like" bite, and they're really filling.
8. One muffin has around 200 calories and 2.5 grams of carbohydrates.

Chapter Twenty-Seven

LOW CARB MUFFINS WITH TUNA

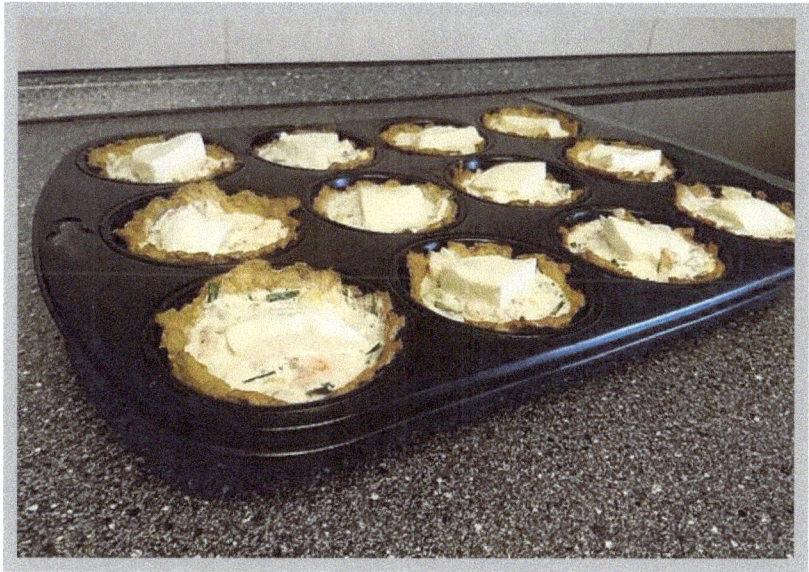

25 MIN.

Simple

. . .

INGREDIENTS

- 1 serving
- 3 cantuna
- 3 egg (s)
- 2 slice / nsmoked salmon
- 1 pck.Crab meat
- 1 garlic cloves)
- 1 spring onion (noun)
- ½ cupcreme fraiche cheese
- 2 tbspcream cheese
- 1 tbspchives
- 1 ballmozzarella
- Salt and pepper
- Lemon juice

PREPARATION

1. Approximate working time: 25 minutes
2. Time to cook/bake: approx. 25 minutes
3. Approximate total time: 50 minutes
4. Drain and pinch the tuna a little first. After whisking the eggs, combine them with the tuna. Fill muffin tins halfway with the batter.
5. Bake for about 10 minutes at 180 degrees in a hot oven.
6. Season with pepper, salt, and lemon juice after chopping the remaining ingredients. Fill the tuna muffins with the mixture after it has cooled for a few minutes and bake at 180 degrees until the perfect browning is achieved.

Chapter Twenty-Eight

LOW CARB PROTEIN MUFFINS

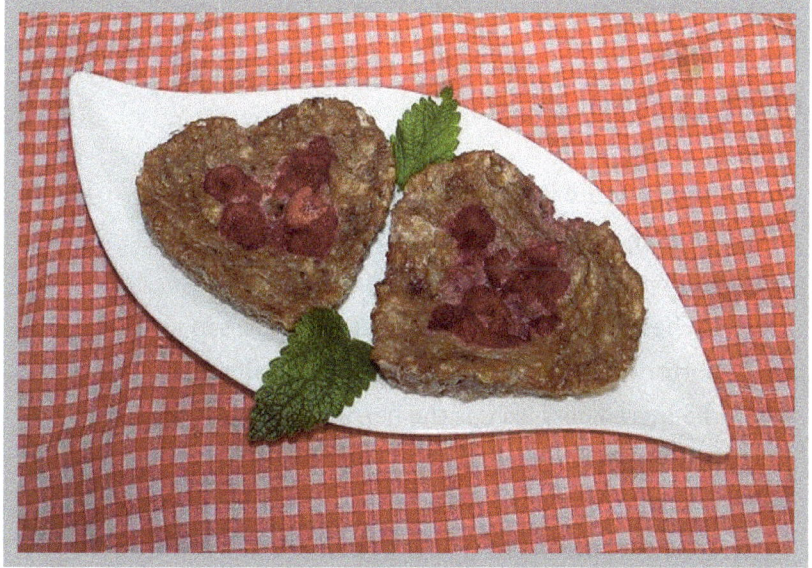

10 MIN.

Normal

. . .

INGREDIENTS

- 1 serving
- 2 banana (noun)
- 50 g protein powder (whey), taste of your choice
- 50 g ground almonds
- 2 egg (s)
- 100 ml milk
- 150 glowfat quark
- 1 tbspcocoa
- 1 teaspoon cinnamon
- 1 teaspoon baking powder
- 200 graspberries

PREPARATION

1. Approximate working time: 10 minutes
2. Time to cook/bake: approx. 25 minutes
3. Approximate total time: 35 minutes
4. Preheat the oven to 200 degrees Celsius, top and bottom. To make a smooth batter, whisk together all of the ingredients except the berries. Fill muffin tins halfway with dough and top with raspberries (silicon baking molds work best).
5. Bake the muffins for about 25 minutes at 200 degrees Celsius.

Chapter Twenty-Nine

LOW CARB HAZELNUT VANILLA MUFFINS

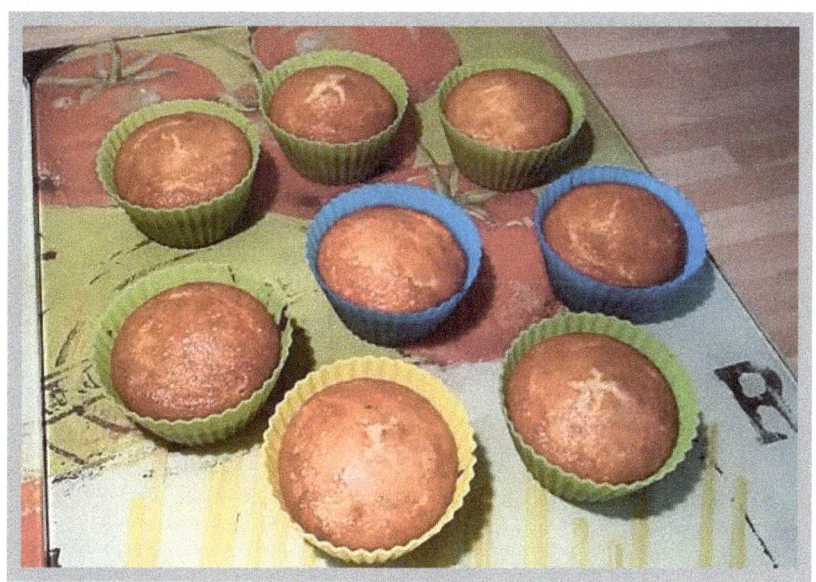

10 MIN.

Simple

. . .

INGREDIENTS

1 servings

- 2 egg (s)
- 50 g mascarpone
- 80 g ground almonds
- 30 g erythritol (sugar substitute)
- 2 tea spoonsbaking powder
- 50 ghazelnuts, chopped
- 2 tbspoil
- 2 vials butter-vanilla flavor

PREPARATION

1. Approximate working time: 10 minutes
2. Approximate cooking / baking time: 20 minutes
3. Approximate total time: 30 minutes
4. Preheat the oven to 140 degrees circulating air or 160 degrees top / bottom heat.
5. In a mixing bowl, combine all ingredients and beat well with a hand mixer. Fill 8 silicone muffin tins halfway with batter. Preheat oven to 350°F and bake for 20 minutes.

www.ingramcontent.com/pod-product-compliance
Lightning Source LLC
Chambersburg PA
CBHW071120030426
42336CB00013BA/2158